Raspberry Ketone Diet Secrets

By Patricia Steele

Exclusive Bonus Resource for Readers of Raspberry Ketone Diet Secrets

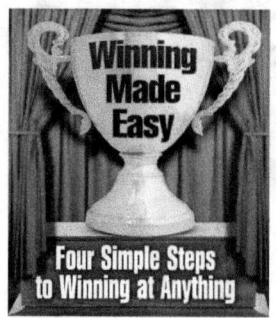

Discover the 4 Steps to Winning Everyday in Every Way in your life!

Learn how you can make money consistently and effortlessly.

Get insider secrets to attracting and keeping your soul mate happy!

Visit http://goo.gl/sQZg9n to claim your above FREE exclusive bonus content.

Introduction

Raspberry ketone-based fat burners are the current supplement "du jour" for weight loss, being touted as a miracle fat burner by numerous celebrities, including the ever-popular Dr. Mehmet Oz. After it was featured on the doctor's show, it was as if the world went crazy and raspberry ketone supplements flew of the shelves. Some retailers being forced to put up signs stating the product in question sold out quickly to avoid problems with disgruntled consumers who hadn't been successful in purchasing the product.

Of course, savvy supplement manufacturers jumped on the train of opportunity and, now, almost every supplement company and their pet dog offers some form of fat-burner based on raspberry ketone. And people keep on buying it in the hopes that it is the miracle Dr. Oz and others have claimed it to be.

It's important to get one thing straight from the get-go. There is no such thing as a miracle weight-loss solution, whether it's a pill, a tea, or some strange ritual involving the full moon and plant sacrifices, that will work without a healthy eating regimen and exercise. If there were, there wouldn't be so many overweight people in the world and it would be selling for a fortune.

Does that mean raspberry ketone doesn't work as a weight-loss supplement? Not at all. It simply means that if you expect to pop a few raspberry ketone pills and watch 25 lbs melt away in a week while you sit on the couch watching your favorite TV show and eat pizza and chips with a chocolate and cookie chaser, then you are going to be very disappointed.

As you will see, raspberry ketone supplements can provide excellent support to your weight loss endeavors but it isn't a miracle fat burner. But you probably already knew that. Yes, it's easy to allow ourselves to believe the hype for a moment because we're all looking for the easy way out. The truth is that there is **no easy way out**. We have to put in some effort but, in a way, it's a good thing, because then we appreciate the results much more.

So, we'll be looking at the potential benefits of raspberry ketone supplementation but it's important that your expectations are realistic. While you might see some results from this compound without changing up your diet and incorporating some incidental activity, they will be minimal and temporary. Therefore, to arm you with all the tools you need to burn off the fat and keep it off, we'll also be looking at the some of the steps you should take to improve your diet and easily incorporate some exercise into your daily routine.

What Is Raspberry Ketone?

Raspberry ketone is a natural phenolic compound – a class of natural organic chemical compounds – that is the main aromatic compound in red raspberries. Contrary to popular belief, this compound can also be found in cranberries and blackberries.

It is used widely in the perfume and cosmetics industry to lend products a fruity smell and is also used as a food additive, to give juices a raspberry flavor, for example. Natural raspberry ketone is quite expensive to produce since it is not that abundant in nature; it takes about 2.5 lbs of raspberries to produce between 1 and 4 mg of this compound. Thus, the natural compound can cost as much as $10,000 per lb.

However, raspberry ketone can also be synthesized using a variety of chemical intermediates. There are various methods to produce this compound but some of them offer as much as a 99% yield. In other words, if 10 lbs of chemicals are used, the result is 9.9 lbs of synthetic raspberry ketone, making it quite cheap. In fact, it only costs a few dollars per pound, which is why most products use the synthetic version.

Raspberry Ketone and Weight Loss

Certain studies conducted on mice and on cells in test tubes have shown that raspberry ketone could accelerate lipolysis, namely the breakdown of fat, as well as prevent fat from accumulating.

One such study was conducted in 2005 at the Eihme University School of Medicine by Morimoto C et al. The study was designed to determine the anti-obese action of raspberry ketone and was conducted on mice. There were two groups of mice. In one case, the mice were fed a high-fat diet with 0.5, 1 or 2% raspberry ketone. The second group was fed a high-fat diet for six weeks after which they were fed the same diet for another five weeks except this time their diet also contained 1% raspberry ketone.

Researchers found that in both cases, when the diet of the mice included this compound, they did not gain weight from the high-fat diet. Weight loss was also observed in the mice whose weight had been increased with a high-fat diet that didn't contain this compound. There was also a significant reduction of fat in the liver.

The study concluded that raspberry ketone seemed to alter how fat is metabolized by activating adiponectin. The latter is a protein hormone that controls various metabolic processes including the processing of fatty acids and the regulation of blood sugar. It seems that the higher the body fat percentage of an individual, the lower the levels of adiponectin in their blood stream.

The discovery of this hormone in the human body is relatively recent and, as such, research is still ongoing. However, it has been found that adiponectin works together with leptin to help regulate body weight. It appears that, when combined, the two hormones improve communication to and from the brain, allowing the body to signal the brain when enough food has been consumed. While there is no clear information as to whether the two hormones must work together to achieve this or have the same effect independently, it has been proven that losing weight can significantly increase the production of this hormone.

Another study conducted in 2010 that was published in Planta Medica supported these findings. Said study was conducted on fat cells in vitro.

The main problem regarding raspberry ketone is that there have been no human clinical trials conducted to prove or disprove its ability to break down fat, which is why many experts are still on the fence regarding this supplement. They state that there have been plenty of other situations in which the effects in vitro and on animals were completely different to the effects of a compound when taken by humans. However, anecdotal evidence supports the efficacy of this compound in helping accelerate weight loss. In most cases, though, significant results were experienced only in conjunction with proper nutrition and exercise.

So, is raspberry ketone effective or not? The reality is that there really is no scientific evidence to support the efficacy of raspberry ketone as a fat burner in humans. Despite this, many doctors recommend their patients take the supplement to see how it will affect them since raspberry ketone is considered a safe substance. Some experts warn, though, that people suffering from certain chronic ailments, such as high blood pressure and asthma, should avoid raspberry ketone due to the fact that its chemical structure is similar to that of a stimulant.

Keep in mind that there have been no studies regarding the side effects of taking raspberry ketone in large doses over a long period of time. In terms of anecdotal evidence, many people reported positive effects but there were some cases in which people experienced a spike in blood pressure, jitteriness and a rapid heartbeat. However, it should be noted that most of the reported side effects were from people who had taken a supplement containing a variety of other ingredients. As such, there is no clear evidence whether raspberry ketone was the cause, or another ingredient or a combination of these ingredients.

So, to put it bluntly, your mileage may vary. But you are likely to see positive results as long as you implement an entire lifestyle change. Otherwise, you are likely to be sorely disappointed.

Remember that you should never start taking a new supplement without consulting your doctor first, especially if you suffer from any chronic conditions or are taking any form of medication.

The Raspberry Ketone Diet: A Three-Pronged Approach

Losing weight and keeping it off is a matter of changing your lifestyle. There is no miracle pill that will help you drop the pounds and look like your favorite celebrity. You need to change your eating habits and incorporate some form of exercise in your daily routine. To boost your weight loss, you can also incorporate various supplements that will help with energy levels as well as potentially increasing your body's ability to burn fat. However, even with these supplements, you won't lose weight if you don't change your diet.

Diet is 75 percent of the equation, exercise another 20 percent and supplementation a mere 5 percent. While diet and exercise are compulsory, you can still lose weight without supplements, though the latter will make life somewhat easier. Now, you can lose weight solely by changing up your diet but your results will be slower in appearing and exercise has many benefits, including reducing the risk of saggy skin. Exercise also helps build your muscles, which is essential to increasing your metabolism. The more muscle mass you have, the more calories you will burn while at rest, making it easier to lose weight and keep it off.

A Lifestyle Change Not a Diet: The Mental Component

If you've ever tried to lose weight before, you're probably already aware that losing weight is more of a mental challenge than anything else. Most people can stick to a diet and an exercise routine as long as they see results but when things start slowing down or they're not seeing the pounds drop as fast as they would like, they give in to food cravings. "It's not working anyway," is the mantra.

So, to lose weight successfully, we need to have the right mindset and realistic expectations because you aren't going to lose all the weight you packed on over five or ten years in one month. It's physically impossible. You can try fad diets or complicated eating plans galore and you might lose an impressive amount of weight at first but as soon as you start eating "normally" you'll pack on the pounds twice as fast. You could put on even more weight.

It makes sense to take a completely different approach to weight loss. Instead of seeing is as a diet, which will come to an end, consider it a lifestyle change to improve your health. You want to look and feel healthy, don't you? You want to have plenty of energy so you can play with your kids, don't you? You want to age gracefully and look forty when you're sixty, don't you? You want to avoid taking tons of medication for various problems from heart disease to high blood pressure, don't you? Well, then, you need to adopt a healthier lifestyle and accept the fact that it's a new of life and not a diet.

That doesn't mean you'll never be able to enjoy a piece of chocolate or a slice of pizza ever again. It simply means these foods should be enjoyed rarely as a treat and not as an everyday occurrence. But while you're main goal is to lose weight, then you need to avoid these foods completely.

Realistic Expectations

If someone could wave a wand and give you a perfectly fit and trim body with abs to die for and buns you could bounce a quarter off of, you'd jump at the chance. Everybody on this planet would. Unfortunately, it doesn't work that way.

It doesn't matter how many diet plans or glossy magazine covers promise to give you the secrets to lose 10 pounds in a week because it doesn't work. Oh, you might lose a substantial amount in your first week but it will be mostly water weight and very little fat. If you have a lot to lose, again, you are likely to see amazing results but in most cases, these plans advocate slashing calories to the point of starvation and it's not a plan that can be maintained for the long-term. It does a lot more harm than good because excessive calorie cutting will slow your metabolism down, making it harder and harder for you to lose weight.

A healthy weight loss goal is to aim for around 2 lbs per week. Any more than that and you are losing water or muscle mass and not fat. Some people, though, won't be able to lose 2 lbs of fat per week if they don't have much to lose.

You have to accept the fact that you are in it for the long haul and commit to a long term plan, no matter how long it takes to get in shape. Remember, the slower you lose the weight, the harder it will be to put it back on. The more time you spend cementing good habits, the easier it will be stick to those habits, which will mean a healthier life and a fitter figure.

Tracking Your Progress

Scales are probably the worst invention known to mankind. That number can play havoc with our minds. We become obsessed with weighing ourselves and get angry when we don't see some progress every day. We want to see results, and we want to see them now. But the scale is a fickle mistress, showing weight fluctuations that can derail even the most dedicated person, even though these fluctuations are usually caused by the natural functions of our body.

It's impossible to put on five pounds of fat in one day, but the scale can make you believe it. So, if you know you are a slave to your scales, you are better off hiding it away at least for the first month and then attempt to weigh yourself no more than once every two weeks, just as a general gauge.

However, if you haven't lost any weight, don't panic. There could be a number of reasons for this including fat loss and muscle gain, which is a good thing. The key is to use a number of methods to track your progress, including body fat measurements – which can be taken with a set of calipers -, the fit of your clothes, before and after pictures and only use the scales once every week or even two.

Whatever you do, though, don't use the scale number as a be-all, end-all because weight can fluctuate for a variety of reasons, including fluid retention, muscle loss or gain and so on and so forth. In fact, women can weigh as much as four or five pounds more during their menstrual cycle because of fluid retention but those pounds disappear as soon as the time of the month is over. Judging your progress via body weight alone is not realistic. You want to focus on losing fat, not water, which is why measuring your body fat will give you a more accurate reading of how well you are doing.

Patience Really Is a Virtue

When it comes to weight loss and improving our health, patience really is a virtue. It will take time but you will learn good habits that will benefit you for the rest of your life. It might take you six months to get to where you want or even longer but in that time you will adopt a healthy lifestyle that will make it much easier for you to maintain your new lean physique. While math does work up to a point, the calories in/calories out principle doesn't work exactly as stated. If it did, we'd be able to drop a consistent number of pounds every week.

There are many other variables that we simply can't calculate realistically, such as activity level, calories burned while at rest and so on. Plus, if that were true, you could eat 1,200 calories worth of burgers, cake and chocolate every day and still lose weight. That doesn't happen.

So, you need to understand that pure math won't work but by adopting clean eating, exercise and introducing a few supplements to rev the metabolic engine up a bit, your body will let go of the weight when its ready but it will let go of it.

Nutrition

Getting your nutrition right is the key to losing weight. It doesn't matter how much you exercise; if you don't change your eating habits, the weight will not come off. Even high-performance athletes who train five hours a day or more can't live on a diet of pizza and chocolate cake. They might not put weight on while they're training but as soon as they take a break, they balloon up. Plus, these foods affect they're performance significantly, which is why they stick to clean, healthy food.

The key to good nutrition is eating whole foods in favor of processed foods, portion control and balanced macronutrients. The balance of macronutrients is important but only up to a point. First, you need to focus on cutting out processed foods and eating cleanly and only once you can say with all certainty that you are eating clean 90% of the time should you consider fiddling with your macronutrient levels.

Portion Control

Portion control is vital to losing weight. Let's be honest, most people eat a lot more than they need to. Portions have gotten exceedingly larger of the past few decades and most meals now consist of over more than 1,000 calories. What's worse is that the quality of the food has dropped, which is why you get hungry a mere hour or two after eating a large meal. By feeding your body processed foods, you aren't giving it all the nutrients it needs and hunger pangs are your body's way of demanding those nutrients.

At first, it can be difficult to practice portion control, especially if you've been skipping breakfast and eating two large meals a day. It will take some self-control but if you eat smaller meals more frequently, you will find it easier to make the right choices and eat less because you aren't as hungry.

Some suggestions to make life easier when it comes to portion control are:

- Use a smaller plate so the meal appears larger;
- Measure out all your food until you can eyeball portion sizes – deluding ourselves is easy;
- Avoid going out to eat until you've mastered the art of portion control;
- When you do go out to eat, either share the entrée with your partner or ask for half of it to be put in a doggie bag before you start to eat.

It will take a while for your body to adjust but as long as you're giving it quality food and are eating the right number of calories, your body will adjust.

Whole Foods

If you want to improve your health and lose weight, you have to avoid processed foods at all costs. In fact, it's a bit difficult to even refer to processed foods as food because most of these products read like a chemical experiment! Even foods that advertise they are all-natural always contain some ingredient that should belong in a laboratory. Most processed foods are empty calories in the best case scenario and downright poison in the worst.

We've basically allowed our taste buds to be trained by large corporations so they can make a larger profit while our waistlines expand. No, it's not completely their fault. It's mainly ours. If we didn't buy and eat the stuff, they wouldn't have a market and wouldn't manufacture the products they do.

You'll find many processed foods contain sugar in one form or another and that includes savory foods that shouldn't include any form of sweetener. But it's been discovered that sugar is addictive so the more sugar a product contains, the more we want to eat. If you look at the ingredient list of the same products from thirty years ago, you will find they contained a fraction of the sugar they do today.

And that's just sugar. Then there's the starch used to bulk up so called meat products. Notice no one actually says meat. It's a meat product. Take chicken nuggets. Do you think a box of frozen chicken nuggets is actually made from meat and nothing but? Unfortunately, no. In many cases, it's a sludge made from leftover chicken bits (including carcasses) that couldn't be used anywhere else, ground down to a paste, and then bulked up with starches and various additives to give them flavor.

So, the first step to a healthier life style and weight loss is to forego processed foods completely and buy fresh, whole foods. You'll find that your taste buds will adapt quickly and, after eating whole foods for a while, you will actually find processed foods unpalatable, especially those containing tons of sugar.

Calories

The age-old question: do calories matter? Unfortunately, they do. You have to burn more than you eat to lose weight but the good news is that most people eat too few calories when they are dieting. Yes, you need to eat less to lose weight but if you eat too little for an extended period of time, your weight loss will grind to a halt and it will be easier for you to regain the weight.

One of the reasons for this is that a drastic reduction in caloric intake has been shown to inhibit leptin secretion. Leptin is a hormone that maintains a balance of energy in the body and regulates hunger. This is achieved by inhibiting the effects of neuropeptide Y – a stimulant that promotes the need to feed, by inhibiting anandamide, which is also a feeding stimulant and by increasing the production of a-MSH, which suppresses the appetite.

It has been found that if there is no leptin present, feeding becomes uncontrolled and relentless. Conversely, in healthy individuals, if leptin is present, the need to eat is reduced. Leptin basically tells the body it has sufficient fat stores and food is not required, so the appetite is reduced. By taking in too few calories, the amount of leptin secreted is reduced, which leads to hunger pangs.

While you might think this isn't anything to worry about, in reality, hormones always win. No matter how much willpower you have, if your body is screaming that you need food, you will eventually give in.

Another problem with a low calorie intake is that your metabolism will start slowing down. Basically, the body is designed to be efficient. This means that over the long term, if your body is only getting 1,000 calories per day, for example, it will hold on to the fat stores it has for as long as possible and begin slowing down or even shutting down certain systems so you can survive on the lower number of calories. The first to go is the libido and reproductive functions. This is why many women who have been on a very low calorie diet for a while will find their menstrual cycle grinds to a halt.

So, how many calories do you need per day? There are many calorie calculators online but, unfortunately, they can't take into account individual factors, such as activity level, exercise, metabolism and more.

A better way to figure out the perfect calorie level for you is to start eating 10 times your body weight in pounds. So, if you weigh 200 lbs, for example, you would start off with 2,000 calories per day. Eat for two weeks at that level and if you lose weight, then stick to that level. You want to create a deficit but not one that is so great that it inhibits the production of leptin and causes you to go into "starvation mode". If you are maintaining, decrease your caloric intake by 250 calories and eat at that level for two weeks and see what happens.

This is a trial and error approach but it will give you a better idea of what will work for you personally than any of the one-size-fits-all calorie calculators online. Another option that will give you a more accurate number is to use the BodyMedia FIT Armband. You wear it throughout the day and it will show you how many calories you burned. Once you have that figure, it's much easier to calculate how many calories you should be consuming to maintain and then to create a safe deficit.

A good rule of thumb, however, is to never drop below your BMR. Keep in mind that you need to recalculate your BMR as you lose weight.

BMR Formula

Women: BMR = 655 + (4.35 x weight in pounds) + (4.7 x height in inches) – (4.7 x age in years)
Men: BMR = 66 + (6.23 x weight in pounds) + (12.7 x height in inches) - (6.8 x age in years)

Macronutrients

The three main macronutrients are protein, fat and carbohydrates. While only protein and fat are absolutely essential, a well-balanced nutrition plan should include all three.

Fat

Fat should be the first macronutrient we talk about simply because it really is essential to the human body but many people are terrified of it. They think that eating fat will make them fat, which is absolutely not true.

Firstly, fat is essential for normal growth and development. It provides the body with energy, protects organs, maintains cell membranes and improves the body's ability to absorb and process nutrients. It also helps the body burn fat, which is why it is a good idea to get one third of your overall calories from fat.

Most of the fat in your diet should come from unsaturated sources because they have a lot of nutrients. These fats, namely monounsaturated fatty acids and polyunsaturated fatty acids, remove LDL cholesterol from your arteries and improve the functioning of your heart, which also help to burn more calories without having to reduce your caloric intake.

When you severely limit your intake of fat, you are making it harder for your body to burn fat. A group of researchers at Washington University School of Medicine in St. Louis explained it like this: "old" fat that is stored in the belly, thighs and butt can't be burned efficiently if there is no "new" fat present, which signals the body that it can get rid of the old fat.

Fat also helps keep you full for longer because it isn't as easy to digest as carbohydrates or proteins. According to the Mayo Clinic, monounsaturated fatty acids help to stabilize blood sugar levels, which means that you won't be hungry right after eating a meal. A study conducted at the University of Navarra in Spain found that people who ate a diet high in omega-3 fatty acids felt fuller right after dinner and for two hours longer than people who ate low levels of these fatty acids. In other words, if you include fat in your diet you are more likely to stick to your good eating habits than if you were to exclude it.

A study conducted in 2011 published in Clinical Science also found that polyunsaturated fatty acids can help to increase protein concentration in the body and grow muscular cells. Increasing muscle mass means increasing the number of calories you burn at rest, in other words you are revving up your metabolism.

Therefore, if you want to be healthy and lose weight, you have to include fat in your diet. You especially should avoid low-fat, no-fat products, which are usually loaded up with sugar and sodium to give the food flavor. Fat gives food flavor and when you remove it, you are left with something completely tasteless, which is why manufacturers add sugar and sodium in large quantities. In other words, you are giving up an essential macronutrient for sugar, which is definitely something you should be avoiding.

Good sources of healthy fats include avocadoes, olives and olive oil, eggs, nuts and seeds and, of course, meat such as chicken and fish and lean cuts of beef, pork and lamb.

Protein

You might be surprised to learn that most people eat too little protein. Protein is the essential building block of the body and eating more of it can help stimulate your metabolism, reduce recovery time after exercise, increase muscle mass and reduce body fat according to a study conducted at the School of Sport and Exercise Sciences at the University of Birmingham in the UK in 2010.

So, exactly how much protein should you be eating to lose weight? Generally, a good recommendation is between 1 and 1.25 grams of protein per pound of lean body mass. So, if you weigh 180 lbs and have 35% body fat, your lean muscle mass is 117 lbs, which means you should be eating between 117 and 146 grams of protein per day.

Carbohydrates
Carbohydrates have been the center of attention for a long time with various "magic formulas" being sold to the public, including low and high carbohydrate eating plans and everything in between. The fact is that completely eliminating carbs is not necessary for most people to lose weight but some form of restriction is necessary.

Carbs raise blood sugar levels, which releases insulin. If there are high levels of insulin in your system, fatty acids cannot be released, so insulin levels need to be managed for fat loss to occur. The simplest way to achieve this is by limiting carbs.

A good rule of thumb is to eliminate simple carbohydrates from processed foods, such as white bread, refined sugar, syrups and soft drinks. You should also limit your intake of simple carbs from natural sources such as milk and dairy products as well as fruit.

Also, try to eat most of your carbs early in the day, when your insulin sensitivity is at its highest. Additionally, carbs should always be eaten as part of a meal that contains protein, fat and fiber. Since they are used to fuel high-intensity exercise, make sure to include them in meals before and after your workout.

Most vegetables can be eaten without restriction due to their high levels of fiber and low carb levels. You want to include one to two servings of vegetables with every meal. This, however, does not include starchy vegetables.

Some examples of vegetables you can eat without restriction include:

- Spinach, collard greens, cabbage, swiss chard, kale
- Broccoli, cauliflower, Brussels sprouts
- Carrots
- Bell peppers
- Asparagus
- Zucchini
- Cucumber, celery
- Mushrooms
- Lettuce
- Tomatoes

How Often Should I Eat?

Meal frequency is not as important as you might think, as long as you are getting all the calories you need. Some nutritionists suggest five meals per day, while others advocate intermittent fasting, which involves having one or two meals per day at the most. All these approaches work but different things work for different people.

For example, you might not be able to eat five meals a day because you can't eat three meals at work. So, three or four meals per day might be a better option for you. Conversely, you might find yourself starving for half the day if you try to eat only one meal per day. It can also be difficult to get all the calories you need in one sitting as you are likely to feel full long before you've had all your calories.

It's a good idea to eat as many small meals per day as you can simply because you won't be as hungry between meals. Some experts claim that it's a good way to rev up your metabolism since your body is receiving fuel throughout the day. Others, though, have seen great results with intermittent fasting. The best solution is the one that works for you as long as you stick to the rule that every meal includes a protein, one or two servings of veggies and a source of healthy fats, such as avocado, olive oil, nuts or seeds.

What to Drink?

Your body is made up of more than 60% water, which means that you need to drink water and plenty of it. A good rule of thumb is to drink at least eight 8-oz glasses of water per day, though some experts recommend as much as a gallon. You want to drink water because it helps you lose fat and assists almost every biological function and chemical reaction in your body. So, forget the diet sodas and flavored drinks and stick to water.

Don't worry, though, you won't have to give up your cup of coffee. In fact, coffee has been shown to reduce the risk of heart disease and other inflammatory diseases. There is also evidence to suggest people who drink coffee are at less risk of developing type II diabetes. Coffee also contains caffeine, cholorogenic acid and quinides which help in fat loss through thermogenesis, increased fat oxidation and a reduction in insulin levels.

Tea and herbal infusions are also good options if you want to change things up.

Exercise

While diet is the most important aspect of weight loss, an exercise program can ensure you succeed because it creates the perfect environment to ensure you are losing fat and not just weight. However, certain types of exercise are more effective than others.

High Intensity Training

When you exercise, you should be pushing yourself to the limit. Of course, you shouldn't do this every day because your body needs a break but at least three times per week is a good idea if you want to lose weight.

High intensity training is important because of the after burn effect known as EPOC, or Excess Post-Exercise Oxygen Consumption. During exercise, oxygen is used to fuel the muscles, which is why you breathe harder while working out. This leads to an oxygen deficit, which needs to be refilled after you finish exercising to ensure proper oxygenation of the blood. Additionally, oxygen and fuel is required to bring your heart rate back to normal, replenish muscle glycogen and for cellular repair. The fuel is, of course, fat. Fatty acids are mobilized to help with recovery.

Exercising at higher levels of intensity has also been shown to be more effective at reducing fat than endurance training, even if fewer calories were burned, according to a study conducted at the Physical Activity Sciences Laboratory of Laval University in Canada.

Strength Training

Strength training is an essential component of any weight loss program because strength training is what really burns the fat, not cardio. It's essential because it helps you build and maintain muscle while you are in a caloric deficit. Otherwise, if you are only doing cardio, your body has no reason to hold on to the muscle and will begin to break it down and use it for energy.

Muscle tissue is vital because one pound of muscle burns 5.67 calories per day, compared to 1.98 calories that a pound of fat burns. It might not seem all that much but if you add 10 pounds of muscle that means you will be burning 56.7 calories per day more. So, that works out to 1,700 calories per month or 20,695 calories per year burned or 6 lbs of fat lost per year without you having to do anything else.

Many women are afraid of strength training because they are afraid that lifting weights will make them bulk up. It doesn't work like that. Firstly, women don't have enough testosterone in their bodies to make them bulk up like men. Secondly, it takes a lot of hard work to put on muscle. It can take as long as a year of heavy training to put on ten pounds of muscle. As long as you keep your diet in check and aren't lifting weights six hours per day, you will not bulk up.

Supplementation

Supplements work but they will have very little effect if you haven't gotten your diet and exercise in order. They won't make up for poor eating habits and inactivity. The fact is that you don't need supplements to lose weight but they can provide support for a good diet and exercise program.

Raspberry Ketone Supplements

There are many raspberry ketone supplements on the market and you have to be careful what you buy. It's generally recommended that you buy supplements that contain only natural raspberry ketone. There are a variety of supplements that also contain other ingredients, which you might want to avoid.

Some experts recommend at least 100 mg of raspberry ketone per day, while others suggest a minimum of 500 mg is required for any real benefits. The best option is to start off with 100 mg and then increase the dosage slowly if you find you aren't gaining any benefits.

Top 10 Tips for Increased Success

The following tips can help you on your weight loss journey. These tips come from people who have lost more than fifty pounds.

1. **Drink Water.** Just by switching over to water and giving up sugary sodas, many people saw tremendous weight loss. You probably don't realize exactly how many calories you are consuming with your four-cans-of-Coke a day habit.

2. **Log Everything You Eat.** Most people have no idea exactly how many calories they consume and by keeping a log of everything you eat, you'll gain better perspective and understand what happens when you eat too much.

3. **Count Calories.** Yes, it's boring and tedious but it's highly effective because it keeps you honest and keeps things in perspective.

4. **Don't Think Diet.** The best weight loss plan is one that suits your lifestyle. Once you discover the perfect fit for you, it will become a way of life rather than something you do for a few months and then go back to "normal".

5. **Consistency Is Key.** No one is perfect and you are bound to make mistakes. But to succeed you need to continue on your journey. Most people who have managed to lose a lot of weight eat healthily at least 90% of the time and don't let the 10% derail them from their plans.

6. **Make a Plan.** Most people make mistakes because they didn't plan for their new lifestyle. That means planning your meals, doing the grocery shopping in advance and even cooking your meals ahead of time.

7. **Small Changes.** Trying to overhaul your life in one go is a recipe for disaster. Instead, people who made small changes consistently found it easier to stick to their new lifestyle. So, change one thing from today and continue making changes consistently.

8. **Become Active.** Anyone who has lost more than fifty pounds did so by adding in some form of physical activity. Find something you enjoy and do it regularly. But you have to push yourself otherwise you are wasting your time.

9. **Get Started.** Don't put it off another day, week or month. Get started right away. The longer you wait, the longer it will take for you to get results.

10. **Do It For You.** You need to focus on yourself and decide to lose weight for yourself and no one else. You are more likely to succeed if you do it because you want to rather than because someone pushed you into it.

Conclusion

While there is some anecdotal evidence that raspberry ketone can be an effective fat burner, there are only a few studies on mice and fat cells in vitro to support this from a scientific viewpoint. However, sufficient people have reported some very positive results to make it worth using as a supplement to add to an effective diet and exercise plan that works for you.

Remember, though, that just taking raspberry ketone supplements alone will not help you lose weight. However, in conjunction with a healthy nutrition plan and an exercise program, they can certainly improve your results and help you lose weight much faster. But before you can experience results like that, you've got to get started.

Take Action Today!

BONUS CONTENT PREVIEW OF THE SPANISH EDITION

Introducción

Los quemadores de grasa a base de cetonas de frambuesas son el actual suplemento " du jour " para bajar de peso, estos se promocionan como un quemador de grasa milagroso por varias celebridades, incluyendo el siempre popular Dr. Mehmet Oz. Después de que fue presentado en el programa del doctor, era como si el mundo se volviera loco y los suplementos de cetona de frambuesa volaron de los estantes. Algunos minoristas fueron obligados a poner carteles donde indicaban que el producto en cuestión se había agotado rápidamente para evitar problemas con los consumidores descontentos que no habían logrado tener éxito al tratar de adquirir el suyo.

Por supuesto, los fabricantes de suplementos inteligentemente se subieron al tren de oportunidades y, ahora, casi todas las empresas de suplementos y sus perros ofrecen algún tipo de quemador de grasa a base de cetona de frambuesa. Y la gente lo sigue comprando con la esperanza de que sea el milagro que el Dr. Oz y otros han afirmado que es.

Es importante dejar una cosa bien claro desde el principio. No hay tal cosa como una solución milagrosa para bajar de peso, si se trata de una píldora, un té, o algún extraño ritual que implica la luna llena y sacrificios de plantas, que funcionará sin un régimen de alimentación saludable y ejercicio. Si la hubiera, no habría tantas personas con sobrepeso en el mundo y se estaría vendiendo por una fortuna.

¿Eso significa que la cetona de frambuesa no funciona como un suplemento para bajar de peso? No, en absoluto. Simplemente significa que si usted espera en bajar 25 libras en una semana sólo tomando un par de píldoras de cetona de frambuesa, mientras que usted está sentado en el sofá viendo su programa favorito de televisión y comiendo pizza y patatas fritas con un chocolate y galletas entonces usted va a salir muy decepcionado.

Como usted verá, los suplementos de cetona de frambuesa pueden proporcionar un excelente apoyo a sus esfuerzos para perder peso, pero no es un quemador de grasa milagroso. Pero es probable que eso ya lo sabías. Sí, es fácil dejarnos llevar por un momento porque todos estamos buscando el camino más fácil. La verdad es que no hay una salida fácil. Tenemos que poner un cierto esfuerzo, pero, en cierto modo, es una buena cosa, porque entonces apreciamos mucho más los resultados.

Por lo tantoestaremos viendo los posibles beneficios de los suplementos de cetona de frambuesa, pero es importante que sus expectativas sean realistas. Mientras que usted verá algunos resultados de este compuesto sin cambiar su dieta e incorporar alguna actividad incidental, serán mínimos y temporales. Por lo tanto, para proporcionarle todas las herramientas que necesita para quemar la grasa y mantenerse en forma, vamos a ver también en algunos de los pasos que debe seguir para mejorar su dieta y fácilmente incorporar algo de ejercicio en su rutina diaria.

¿Qué es la cetona de frambuesa?

La cetona de frambuesa es un compuesto fenólico natural - una clase de compuestos químicos orgánicos naturales - que son los compuestos aromáticos principales en las frambuesas rojas. Contrario a la creencia popular, este compuesto también se puede encontrar en los arándanos y moras.

Se utiliza ampliamente en la industria de la perfumería y la cosmética para darle a los productos un olor afrutado y también se utiliza como aditivo alimentario, para darle sabor frambuesa a los jugos, por ejemplo. La cetona de frambuesa natural es bastante cara de producir, ya que no es que abundante en la naturaleza, sino que se requieren 2,5 libras de frambuesas para producir entre 1 y 4 mg de este compuesto. Por lo tanto, el compuesto natural puede costar hasta $ 10.000 por libra

Sin embargo, la cetona de frambuesa también se puede sintetizar usando una variedad de productos químicos intermedios. Existen varios métodos para producir este compuesto, pero algunos de ellos ofrecen hasta un 99% de rendimiento. En otras palabras, si se utilizan 10 libras de productos químicos, el resultado es 9,9 libras de cetona de frambuesa sintética, por lo que abarata bastante el precio. De hecho, sólo cuesta unos pocos dólares por libra, por lo que la mayoría de los productos utilizan la versión sintética.

La Cetona de Frambuesa y la Pérdida de Peso

Ciertos estudios realizados en ratones y en células en tubos de ensayo han demostrado que la cetona de frambuesa podría acelerar la lipólisis, es decir, la descomposición de la grasa, así como evitar la acumulación de grasa.

Uno de estos estudios se llevó a cabo en el 2005 en la Escuela de Medicina de la Universidad Eihme por Morimoto C et al. El estudio fue diseñado para determinar la acción anti - obesidad de la cetona de frambuesa y se llevó a cabo en ratones. Hubo dos grupos de ratones. En un caso, los ratones fueron alimentados con una dieta alta en grasas con 0,5, 1 o 2 % de cetona de frambuesa. El segundo grupo fue alimentado con una dieta alta en grasas durante seis semanas después de que fueron alimentados con la misma dieta durante cinco semanas, salvo en esta ocasión su dieta también contenía un 1 % de cetona de frambuesa.

Los investigadores encontraron que en ambos casos, cuando la dieta de los ratones incluía este compuesto, no aumentaron de peso usando esta dieta alta en grasas. La pérdida de peso también se observó en los ratones cuyo peso había aumentado con una dieta alta en grasa que no contienen este compuesto. También hubo una reducción significativa de grasa en el hígado.

El estudio concluyó que la cetona de frambuesa parecía alterar la cantidad de grasa que se metaboliza mediante la activación de la adiponectina. Esta última es una hormona proteica que controla varios procesos metabólicos, incluyendo el procesamiento de ácidos grasos y la regulación de azúcar en la sangre. Parece que cuanto mayor es el porcentaje de grasa corporal de un individuo, más bajos serán los niveles de adiponectina en su torrente sanguíneo.

El descubrimiento de esta hormona en el cuerpo humano es relativamente reciente y, como tal, la investigación todavía sigue en curso. Sin embargo, se ha descubierto que la adiponectina funciona junto con la leptina para ayudar a regular el peso corporal. Parece ser que, cuando se combinan, las dos hormonas mejoran la comunicación hacia y desde el cerebro, permitiendo que el cuerpo de la señal al cerebro cuando suficiente comida ha sido consumida. Si bien no hay información suficiente en cuanto a si las dos hormonas deben trabajar juntas para lograr esto o que tengan el mismo efecto de forma independiente, se ha demostrado que la pérdida de peso puede aumentar significativamente la producción de esta hormona.

Otro estudio realizado en el 2010 que fue publicado en la Planta Medica ha apoyado estos hallazgos. Dicho estudio se llevó a cabo en las células de grasa en vitro.

El principal problema con respecto a la cetona de frambuesa es que no se han realizado ensayos clínicos en humanos probar o refutar su capacidad para descomponer la grasa corporal, por lo que muchos expertos están todavía a la defensiva con respecto a este suplemento. Ellos afirman que ha habido un montón de otras situaciones en las que los efectos in vitro y en animales salieron completamente diferentes a los efectos de un compuesto cuando fueron tomados por los seres humanos. Sin embargo, la evidencia anecdótica apoya la eficacia de este compuesto para ayudar a acelerar la pérdida de peso. En la mayoría de casos, sin embargo, los resultados significativos se experimentaron sólo en combinación de una nutrición adecuada y ejercicio.

Por lo tanto, ¿la cetona de frambuesa es efectiva o no? La realidad es que realmente no hay evidencia científica que apoye la eficacia de la cetona de frambuesa como quemador de grasa en humanos. A pesar de ello, muchos médicos recomiendan a sus pacientes tomar el suplemento para ver si hay algún efecto ya que la cetona de frambuesa es considerada una sustancia segura. Algunos expertos advierten, sin embargo, que las personas que sufren de ciertas enfermedades crónicas, como presión arterial alta y el asma, deben evitar la cetona de frambuesa, debido al hecho de que su estructura química es similar a la de un estimulante.

Tenga en cuenta que no se han realizado estudios sobre los efectos secundarios de tomar la cetona de frambuesa en grandes dosis durante un largo período de tiempo. En términos de evidencia anecdótica, muchas personas reportaron efectos positivos, pero hubo algunos casos en que las personas han experimentado un aumento en la presión arterial, temblores y un ritmo cardíaco acelerado. Sin embargo, cabe señalar que la mayoría de los efectos secundarios observados fueron de personas que habían tomado un suplemento que contiene una variedad de otros ingredientes. Como tal, no hay evidencia clara si la cetona de frambuesa fue la causa, o fue otro ingrediente o una combinación de estos ingredientes.

Así que, para decirlo sin rodeos, sus resultados pueden variar. Pero es probable que vea resultados positivos, siempre y cuando se implemente un cambio completo de estilo de vida. De lo contrario, es probable que sea una gran decepción.

Recuerde que nunca debe comenzar a tomar un nuevo suplemento sin consultar primero a su médico, especialmente si usted sufre de alguna condición crónica o está tomando algún tipo de medicamento.